THE EFFECT OF MEDITATION AND RELAXATION ON INDIVIDUALS DIAGNOSED WITH LONG-TERM SCHIZOPHRENIA

THE EFFECT OF MEDITATION AND RELAXATION ON INDIVIDUALS DIAGNOSED WITH LONG-TERM SCHIZOPHRENIA

Anthea Morne, RN, Ph.D, LMHC, CASAC

WESTBOW
PRESS®
A DIVISION OF THOMAS NELSON
& ZONDERVAN

WestBow Press books may be ordered through booksellers or by contacting:

WestBow Press
A Division of Thomas Nelson & Zondervan
1663 Liberty Drive
Bloomington, IN 47403
www.westbowpress.com
1 (866) 928-1240

This book is a work of non-fiction. Unless otherwise noted, the author and the publisher make no explicit guarantees as to the accuracy of the information contained in this book and in some cases, names of people and places have been altered to protect their privacy.

ISBN: 978-1-9736-2153-9 (sc)
ISBN: 978-1-9736-2154-6 (hc)
ISBN: 978-1-9736-2152-2 (e)

Library of Congress Control Number: 2018902457

Print information available on the last page.

WestBow Press rev. date: 5/11/2018

CONTENTS

PREFACE: MY OWN PATH TO MEDITATION AND RELAXATION

For five decades I served as a registered professional nurse. My professional nursing training began at an early age on the small island of Dominica, West Indies. Shortly after completing my initial nursing training I immigrated to the United States to continue my nursing career and further my nursing education.

Early on, I took advantage of opportunities to work in various healthcare fields. I studied maternity and child nursing, medical and surgical practice, pediatric care and neonatal pediatric care, geriatric care, and alcohol and other drug detoxification services. For the last thirty years of my career, my primary focus has been psychiatry. Specifically, working with individuals diagnosed with long-term schizophrenia.

In 2002, I had the opportunity to facilitate a weekly group session for individuals living with long term schizophrenia. Prior to accepting this role I reflected on my experiences and observations over the years. I thought of the effective best practices used to engage individuals living with long term schizophrenia. It was not so much based on science, but most often on demeanor. I thought of my colleagues and mentors that effectively de-escalated crisis, promoted feelings of safety amongst the patients and most importantly made the patients feel like they mattered. Their demeanors were patient focused, compassionate, intuitive and kind. Their interactions promoted a calmness that resulted in positive outcomes. I decided to mirror their practices by promoting the use of meditation and relaxation techniques in a group setting.

Evidence shows the use of meditation and relaxation techniques in a group setting can produce positive outcomes for persons diagnosed with long term schizophrenia. Group sessions would be conducted in conjunction with a prescribed medication regimen and other prescribed therapeutic interventions.

To my knowledge, I am the first healthcare professional in my facility to commence a meditation and relaxation group for individuals diagnosed with long term schizophrenia. The onset proved to be challenging, however over time the therapeutic relationship improved to the point participants anticipated and requested to attend group. Group sessions occurred every Sunday for six years.

ACKNOWLEDGMENTS

I must first thank my God for giving me the strength, courage, and wisdom to work hard to attain my goals. I am indebted to my brother, Anthony, my mentor, who stood by my side and encouraged me to pursue my passion and share my experiences. I thank my daughter, Johanne, for her continuous support. I wish to say thank you for guidance that I have received from the faculty members of IUGS including Ms. West, Dr. Dorritie, and Dr. Lohmiller. Your support and encouragement will always be remembered. To my deceased husband, Jean Marie, and my parents, Hilton and Veronique Seraphin, thank you for supporting me in spirit.

Anthea

THE BEGINNING
OF LEARNING

My acceptance and knowledge of meditation and relaxation began at an early age. At a young age my learning came in the form of spiritualism. My family raised me with a strong faith in Roman Catholicism. Before going to bed, we knelt and prayed together. It was a time of peaceful reflection. Weekdays, we awoke early to attend 5:30 a.m. church service. I accepted that the opportunity of prayer could create a peaceful space of meditation and relaxation.

Throughout my nursing career I would not only educate patients on the necessary steps to achieve quality physical health. I encouraged patients to focus on their mental and emotional health – strengthened through the learned techniques of meditation and relaxation.

Schizophrenia

Individuals with this diagnosis are often reported to be isolated and unable to form relationships with other people (Mitchell and Black 1995). The Oxford Dictionary describes schizophrenia as, "a long-term mental disorder whose symptoms include inappropriate actions and feelings and withdrawal from reality and fantasy" (2001). In a 1999 overview of schizophrenia from the National Institute of Mental Health, schizophrenia is described as, "a chronic, severe, and disabling brain disease" (Spearing, et al. 1999. 2002).

Schizophrenia is a type of brain disease that interferes with the normal brain functioning. The onset age is defined as between sixteen and twenty-five years. Onset is uncommon after thirty years and very rare after forty years. Schizophrenia affects more men than women aged sixteen to twenty-five years old. From the ages of twenty-five and thirty years, it is more common in women than in men.

Brain diseases like schizophrenia alter the thinking, feeling, understanding, and consciousness. The common symptoms of schizophrenia are difficulty thinking, difficulty interacting with others, inability to carry out responsibilities, and difficulty controlling emotions and expressions appropriately. Thus the disease affects every aspect of the of a person's life, work, social life, and family life.

HOW IS SCHIZOPHRENIA DIAGNOSED?

The criteria for the diagnosis of schizophrenia is well documented in the *Diagnostic and Statistical Manual of Mental Disorders* (DSM), which is used by mental health clinicians for proper diagnosis. The DSM also claims that schizophrenia is a disturbance that lasts for at least six months and includes at least one month of actual phase symptoms, such as delusions, hallucinations, disorganized speech, and grossly disorganized or catatonic behavior. In the *Live Search Health Article-Schizophrenia,* five subtypes of schizophrenia are cited.

Catatonic Type. Considered to be one of the major types of schizophrenia, this illness is characterized by marked motor abnormalities, including motored immobility (i.e., catalepsy or stupor) (DSM-IV 1994). Some of the symptoms may include decreased sensitivity, inability to take care of personal needs, and negative feelings (Schizophrenic Information on Health Line 2005–2009).

Disorganized Thoughts Type. This type may include disorganized speech, disorganized behavior, or flat and inappropriate affect (DSM-IV 1994). Disorganized schizophrenia, or hebephrenic, is one of the subtypes of schizophrenia in which there is an extreme expression of disorganization syndrome. Other symptoms include hallucinations, delusions, lack of spontaneous movement, blunting of emotions, and poor speech. Disorganized schizophrenia is characterized by incoherent and illogical thoughts in words as well in behavior.

Paranoid Type. The essential feature is the presence of prominent delusions or auditory hallucinations. The individual suspects that others are plotting to harm them without any basis. The individual also has unjustified doubts about the loyalty or trustworthiness of friends, family, and associates (DSM-IV 1994). People with paranoid subtype are more functional in their performance and more into engagements and relationships with people as compared to the other types of schizophrenia. People who suffer from this subtype usually do not exhibit any clear symptoms until later in life, or they achieve the highest level of functioning before the onset of the disease.

Residual Type. This form of schizophrenia has no positive symptoms. There are no delusions or hallucinations, disorganized speech, or catatonic symptoms (Oxford Dictionary of Psychology 2006). This is a transition between a full-blown episode and a complete remission. Residual schizophrenia may be present for many years with or without exacerbation (DSM-IV 1994).

Undifferentiated Type. This major type of schizophrenia is similar to the residual type. There are no signs or symptoms characteristic of catatonic, disorganized, or paranoid schizophrenia (Oxford Dictionary of Psychology 2006). Evidence of the disturbance is indicated by the presence of negative symptoms such as odd beliefs and unusual perceptual experiences (DSM-IV 1994).

WHO ATTENDED THE GROUP SESSION?

Group attendance ranged from eighteen to twenty patients. The majority of participants are male. Individuals were diagnosed with one of the five subtypes of schizophrenia noted above. On most occasions more than ninety percent of group participants were observed to be alert, oriented to person, place and time, and have little or no evidence of agitation or somatic concerns. For those participants unable to actively participate, due to presenting symptoms of their diagnosis interventions included, verbal redirection, relocation to a less stimulating environment.

Of the group participants fifty percent met the criteria for the residual type of schizophrenia, while twenty percent met the criteria for undifferentiated type (interestingly for this subtype, there was no evidence of psychomotor agitation and an absence of auditory and visual hallucinations). An estimated twenty percent met criteria for paranoid type and undifferentiated type. Ten percent met criteria for disorganized type. In this type, there was some impairment of cognition and poor insight, but there was no behavioral effect.

An estimated 90 percent of group participants presented

with a long history of mental illness (exceeding thirty years). The remaining 10 percent had suffered from mental illness for less than thirty years. Participants' ages ranged from forty-nine to seventy-two. Individuals volunteered to participate with the understanding that if at any time they felt uncomfortable or began to feel anxious about their participation, they were free to leave the meditation room space quietly and later return if they wished to continue with the meditation.

PROMOTION AND SET UP OF THE GROUP SETTING

otice of the Group Session was publicly posted on a bulletin board in the hallway of the care unit. The posting announced a meditation and relaxation group in the dayroom every Sunday evening at 7:30 p.m. The posting clearly stated that everyone was free to *voluntarily* attend. The posting indicated that further information and/or concerns about the group could be addressed to the facilitator.

Participants were informed that they are welcome to leave the group quietly at any time It is important to acknowledge that it can be extremely difficult, if not impossible, to have individuals diagnosed with long term schizophrenia sit quietly for any period of time without feeling anxious and agitated. However, patients who are not in an acute phase of their mental illness should be able to actively participate in a meditation and relaxation group lasting approximately forty-five to fifty minutes, if a quiet atmosphere is created for them.

To conduct the meditation and relaxation group, the patients are taken to a quiet and spacious room, where they are seated in a circle in straight-backed chairs. A CD player is placed on a table that is covered with a clean white sheet and located at the top of the room. The facilitator is seated near the table while the CD player plays a soft, non-vocal spiritual tune to create a calming and relaxing atmosphere.

This group initially began with twenty participants, consisting of seventeen males and three females, and gradually increased to twenty-eight participants. The session begins with the facilitator asking everyone to sit upright in a relaxing position, with feet on the floor and palms resting upward on their laps in an 'asking' position. The participants are asked to listen and follow the verbal directions that are given. The facilitator proceeds to guide the participants in taking three long, slow, deep breaths, one breath each for the body, mind, and spirit. Participants are then invited to clear their minds of any anxiety, fear, and agitation, and to presently focus only on their wellbeing. These successive deep breaths are repeated several times during the meditation and relaxation session. The participants are guided to remain in a meditative state. They are asked to draw each breath down into each muscle that controls the breathing and to visualize, as the breaths are inhaled, an illumination of the internal organs, followed by an external body radiation with rays of clear white light that will aid in the promotion of healing. As they exhale through the mouth, they will visualize that they are exhaling into the universe the stress, anxiety, fears, and tension that is experienced within their body and mind.

The meditation continues for thirty to forty-five minutes. The participants continue to remain in that meditative state while they are guided by the facilitator to enter into a flower garden, with rays of sunshine filtering through the foliage, and they are guided to listen to the sound of chirping birds. Participants are instructed to raise their eyes up to the sky mentally and visualize a beautiful blue sky with some clouds lazily floating across it, as well as streams of clear water flowing at the four corners of this beautiful flower garden.

The room is filled with a soft and relaxing non-vocal spiritual theme throughout the session. A phrase or mantra, such as *ohm* or *all is well*, is slowly repeated throughout the session. Before the session ends, participants are gently guided to send love and healing energy to loved ones not present in the session. They are instructed to visualize that their loved one is sitting in a chair or resting comfortably in bed. A soft healing blanket is formed visually with rays of beautiful blue color. The participants are guided to send love and healing energy with all the love in their heart to their loved ones. They are reminded that sending love and healing energy to others is a voluntary act for both sender and recipient. If the recipient is not ready to receive, and/or if the sender has no one in mind at the present moment to send the love and healing energy to, they can send it to "Mother Earth," who will take care of that energy. The session ends with participants being guided to mentally give thanks to the spiritual guides who are present and assisting during the session. After closing, participants are asked to remain seated and served refreshments.

EVIDENCE OF THE POSITIVE BENEFITS OF MEDITATION AND RELAXATION

People diagnosed with long term schizophrenia often report feeling intimidated. Research suggests that individuals are better able to control their disease related symptoms by creating an awareness of their surroundings. According to Sohee Park, neuropsychologist of Vanderbilt University, "We are interested to see if teaching can help improve the control over the symptoms of schizophrenia." For such purposes, different therapeutic approaches, such as yoga and dance, have also been proven to work.

Existing research is conclusive that achieving a meditative state can result in decreased stress and anxiety which leads to increased quality of health and living. Meditation promotes a shift of the conscious use of one's mind, rather than being used by one's mind. (Beckwith 2008).

The practice of meditation varies from thoughtful contemplation to inner discipline of consciousness that can often induces profound spiritual enlightenment. In the eastern philosophies, Buddhist and Taoist meditation, meditation is viewed as a way to realize and integrate into every day life certain "external truths," an approach that is particularly valuable in the modern world, which has become fogged by illusion (George 2004). Tranquility and relaxation are the natural norms of the mind, body, and spirit. Meditation and relaxation, can restore natural peacefulness and calmness.

Meditation is a simple, ancient, universal, and natural technique for the development of human potential. This technique requires concentration, effort, and/or suggestion. After receiving initial instruction from a qualified teacher, meditation is practiced by sitting comfortably, with the eyes closed, for fifteen to twenty minutes, twice a day. It is not a religion, a philosophy, or a way of life. At present, more than six million people of all nationalities and culture practice meditation for overcoming stress (Benson 2005).

There are many things in life that lie beyond the reach and control of human beings. However, understanding the theory behind these facets of life can help us take responsibility to create our own state of mind, one in which we feel comfortable so that we can change the rest according to our own benefit. According to Buddhism, this is one of the most important things we need to consider to live a happy and contended life. Buddhism teaches us that this is the antidote, easily available for everyone, to overcome our sorrow, grief, anxiety, fears, and feelings of hatred and confusions. These are the states that move the human living condition toward distress. Meditation is a means to transform the mind, directing it toward the thoughts we want to experience. Buddhist meditation techniques make us practice concentration, clarity, emotional positivity, encouragement, and modifying learning patterns.

Such practices are used to cultivate more positive thoughts, develop good habits for the mind and body, as well as live life positively. With regular exercise, practicing meditation helps us nourish our mind with more powerful and positive thoughts, and the mind becomes deeper, more focused, more peaceful, and more energized. Collectively, these effects bring positive changes in life and transformations that give a new understanding to life.

There are countless meditation practices followed in the Buddhist tradition. In simple terms, we can describe all such practices as "mind trainings," but each one follows a distinct approach. The basic foundation of all of them is to remain in a calm and positive state of mind. The meditation techniques are very simple to learn and understand. However, it is always recommended to learn them from an experienced and reliable trainer or teacher, who can provide guidance on how to apply techniques to overcome problems and can make you understand the key to overcoming difficulties. Most importantly, teachers offer encouragement and inspiration in learning and practicing meditation.

To prepare for meditation, one must sit down and find one's meditation posture, typically a relaxed, upright position. Usually people sit on a cushion with their legs crossed. People who cannot sit like this or who face difficulty sitting down on the floor can kneel or even use a chair. You then close your eyes, relax, and tune your mind to the way you want to feel. It is very important to be sensitive to feelings and experiences, because this is the way positive thoughts are forced into your mind, pulling out negative ones. This is the main practice you need to work on in meditation. It is always good to sit back quietly, relax, and think positively before starting any meditation practice. Some teachers also recommend gentle stretching to slow down and relax. People who practice meditation have been quoted as saying that the benefits of meditation are various and that they help the person experience a deeper sense of being. The mind becomes free of agitation; it remains clam and at peace, quiet and free of negative thoughts. This is what meditation helps you experience.

Meditation is considered one of the essential practices for good mental hygiene. Improvement in the thought process, clarity in thoughts, concentration at work, blossoming of skills, refining of talents, and inner strength and courage make you feel more comfortable at work and even at home. All such healing powers help you to relax, rejuvenate, and create a source of inner energy that keeps you alive and energetic. In today's world, where stress, anxiety, hassle, and fear catch up faster than a person can perceive with one's mind, meditation can be an easily accessible source of luxury. Those who have experienced find it necessary to live a peaceful and happy life.

There are different types of meditation. Examples of meditation used with the group sessions include, passive meditation, Transcendental Meditation (TM), guided meditation, yoga, chi gung, traditional meditation, tai chi, and many more. When the focus is kept on the path of enlightenment in order to obtain some form of effectiveness, by group or individuals, then it can produce positive effects.

In a review related to the integration of meditation in higher education, Shapiro et al. (2008) found that an individual's ability to maintain preparedness and orient attention can be improved with the help of mindfulness meditation. Mindfulness meditation is helpful in reducing stress, depression, and anxiety, and mindfulness meditation supports better regulation of emotional reactions and helps give rise to positive psychological states (Shapiro et al. 2008). An article written the technique of tai chi referred to it as an exercise for mind and body. Brown and Jones (2010) state that people who practice this technique reported that afterward they felt stronger in their legs, more alert, and more focused and relaxed (Brown and Jones 2010).

Holden (2010), a researcher as well as a practitioner of chi gung meditation, in his DVD *Qi Healing Energy Practice for Health and Vitality*, cites the ability of this technique to empower the mind, body, and spirit, which in turn gives one the feeling of being healthier and at the pinnacle of serenity. He also iterates that this meditation must be practiced with gentle rhythmic movements (Holden 2010).

Guided imagery is another alternative option in the field of mindfulness meditation. Practicing this technique enables an individual to release fear, tension, and anxiety. When these feelings are kept in check, the individual becomes able to concentrate in the present and remain in the moment. Luzader (2002), in her CD *Guided Imagery: For Stress Release and Relaxation* cites how this technique of guided imagery can be used to eliminate anxiety and to boost relaxation.

According to Bogart (1991) it is important to take into consideration theories that suggest that meditation leads to cognitive, physiological, and behavioral changes that may produce therapeutic benefits. Theories also affirm ways through which meditation can be considered more than just an exercise of relaxation. It can be considered cognitive and behavioral therapy (Bogart 1991).

Deatherage (1975) conducted studies about the effectiveness of meditation techniques. In these studies, he considered meditation a primary or secondary technique with a range of psychiatric patients. According to Deatherage, meditation can be considered a self-treatment regimen. Meditation, he believes, gives patients knowledge about their own mental processes and preoccupations. It allows one to develop the observer self. Meditation provides the ability to an individual so that mental processes can be shaped or controlled (Deatherage 1975).

Numerous scientific studies document the effectiveness and benefits of Transcendental Meditation at all levels. It increases awareness, creativity, and intelligence. In addition, it provides resistance to stress and reduces anxiety. Meditation is a source of mental clarity, decision-making, and self-esteem. Furthermore, it provides resistance to disease and promotes cardiovascular health together, along with more happiness and peace. Meditation also plays an important role in improving behavior and interpersonal relationships. (Naim 1999).

In the view of Deikman (1982), meditation should not be considered a replacement for therapy; rather, it is an adjunct to it. For patients who are suffering from serious mental illness and for patients who have reached a long-term stage, meditation alone cannot be effective. However, the fact cannot be ignored that when meditation is practiced on a regular basis, it helps by releasing stress, anxiety, and other signs of depression (Deikman 1982).

A study was conducted on 322 patients in which mindfulness-based stress-reduction (MBSR) meditation training was provided for ten weeks. After the completion of the training it was found that MBSR had been effective and played an immense role in reducing the physical, cognitive, and emotional consequences of chronic stress. It can be extracted from various researches that if meditation is used effectively, it produces positive results with regards to stress and other factors of environment. A number of studies that prove that the technique of meditation and relaxation is being practiced in various organizations and has shown to be extremely beneficial (Alexander, Walton, and Johnson 2013).

In Japan, a study was conducted by Johnson (2006) on eight hundred industrial workers. These eight hundred workers took part in a Transcendental Meditation course. Johnson reports that a decrease was noticed in physical complaints, depression, anxiety, neurotic tendencies, insomnia, and somatic complaints.

Another form of meditation that is being practiced by many mental health practitioners and others is the activating of the chakras. According to Tipping (2009), human beings possess a system of energy centers that align vertically in our bodies. These are known as chakras ("wheel" in Sanskrit), which are like vortices of spinning energy. Tipping (2009 noted seven major chakra points used in meditation, which are interrelated. If one chakra point becomes disturbed or blocked, it can upset the functioning of the others—this can manifest itself as emotional feelings of being depressed as well as physical problems, stemming from whichever area is most vulnerable.

Recently, much attention has been given to meditation and relaxation techniques to improve mental as well as physical health. It improves emotional wellbeing, increases immune responses, reduces pain, and fosters spiritual growth. An integrative review of the research related to meditation, spirituality, and the elderly by Deborah A. Lindberg (2005) covered the research conducted for the last twenty-five years on meditation and spirituality, particularly considering the state of health among the elderly suffering from dementia. The results supported the hypothesis that meditation and spirituality promote social and emotional benefits for those elderly who live in isolation. It was also reported that these practices can be implemented in nursing homes to achieve high levels of effectiveness.

Mindfulness is an attribute of the consciousness, believed to promote mental wellbeing. Brown et al. (2003), in the article "The Benefits of Being Present: Mindfulness and Its Role in Psychological Wellbeing," provided a theoretical and empirical examination of mindfulness and the role it can play in psychological wellbeing. The Mindful Attention Awareness Scale (MAAS) measures the level of consciousness to construct wellbeing and enhance self awareness. Quasi-experimental and sampling studies have proven that both the state of mindfulness and disposition regulates behavior and positive emotional states.

Months to years practice of meditation on an intensive level can improve attention and thought processes. A random group was assigned to practice meditation for five days, along with interactive mind and body trainings. The results were a marked increase in control over stress and better attention, which was similar to the control group, which was given relaxation training. The training followed various Chinese practices and other meditation and mindfulness trainings. A control group was also designated, and the experimental group comprised forty undergraduate students. The experimental group was given twenty minutes of integrative training sessions for five days to show improvement in conflict scores on the Attention Network Test. The Mood States Scale showed lower anxiety, fatigue, anger, depression, and high vigor. It was also noted that there was an increase in immune-reactivity and a decrease in stress-related cortisol. Therefore, the results support that meditation does influence the mindfulness and relaxation process (Tang et al. 2007).

The clinical effectiveness of meditation in psychiatric disorders is due to changes in neurobiology. Several researches have been published that provide evidence that the changes produced by meditation on brain and body physiology are evident and effective in the treatment of psychiatric disorders. The main aim of meditation is to eliminate the negative thought process, which prevails over the mind, and advance the mind toward internalized thinking, leading to physical and mental relaxation. All these changes cause stress reduction, enhanced concentration, and psycho-emotional stability. Physiological changes are observed in the autonomic and endocrine functioning. Whole neuro-imaging shows the regions of the brain which control attention. Clinical studies have also shown that meditation is effective in treating the disorders of stress, anxiety, and lack of attention. Still more research needs to be done to confirm the clinical effectiveness of meditative practices and the role they play in the prevention and intervention of mental illness (Rubia 2009).

EFFECTS OF MEDITATION AND RELAXATION INTERVENTIONS ON INDIVIDUALS DIAGNOSED WITH LONG TERM SCHIZOPHRENIA

Beckwith (2008) states that with the help of meditation, one can obtain the transformation one needs for inner peace. It is not easy to defy this assertion, because attaining peace from within requires an individual to be at a powerful moment. We must never forget that meditation is not a cure but a way to spiritual evolution. While it is possible to overstate the results, with reason, and perhaps with the help of someone who has more experience, people can bring everything within their limits. However, it is essential to continue with patience and due diligence (Nelson 1990).

When psychological problems alter the sensitivity to and perception of the surrounding world, people are required to be very careful, considering right away if meditation began before or after the onset of disorders. During periods of stress, those who meditated before can safely continue to do so. However, he must be aware that even if the first impulse may be to detach from a stressful time, this detachment must still be a way for a conscious approach to one's choice of spiritual quest, with the primary purpose being to get out of one's own selfishness and simply learn to live without doing harm to oneself or others. There is a minimum of spiritual need.

If the stressed person forgets meditation and plays sports, exercises, performs relaxation techniques, or does anything else to distract them, this can be good as long as it does not create new problems (Baumeister and Leary 1995).

A US study published in the *Proceedings of the National Academy of Sciences* photographed the effect that this discipline has on the brain, noting a direct action on the medial prefrontal cortex and the posterior cingulated nucleus, whose excessive activation is linked to disorders of attention and some psychiatric diseases, in particular, schizophrenia and autism. Researchers at Yale University observed only among those who practice meditative disciplines for a long time, not among the neophytes. Moreover, it was present even when the "experts" did nothing. Several studies have verified the benefits of this practice, and some types of psychotherapy have begun to exploit its prerogatives. There is a genetic predisposition to the ability to focus, and an unfavorable gene structure cannot be corrected by simply meditating (Gross 1998).

According to a new study on imaging carried out by researchers from Yale University, people who practice meditation, through experience, become capable of controlling areas of the brain associated with 'daydreaming'. Furthermore, according to many scholars of psychiatry, one's ability in meditation is associated with a rise in happiness levels (Salzberg 1995).

In the past, meditation has proven capable of alleviating

a variety of health problems. It is useful to quit smoking and dealing with cancer and even psoriasis. The research team at Yale University conducted the new study using functional magnetic resonance imaging on a group of experienced meditators and a group of beginners who practiced three different meditation techniques (Hick and Bien 2008). Experienced meditators have been shown to reduce activity in brain areas associated with attention disorders and anxiety, as well as in the formation of beta-amyloid plaques characteristic of Alzheimer's disease. The decrease in activity in this area, which corresponds to the medial prefrontal cortex and the posterior cingulated, is observed in experienced meditators regardless of the technique they use. Meditation is essential to the mental health and wellbeing of human beings. However, if people lack integrity in their practice, it could cause them problems. Some people have difficulties such as depression, anxiety, and schizophrenia and believe that meditation is an instant cure for their problems. They begin to meditate, and on some occasions their problems get worse. If people have a problem like this, they should first seek professional help and then devote themselves to meditation. Other people strive to do too much in meditation, without practicing it gradually, step by step. They meditate with too much power for too long, and they run out of steam. However, the majority of problems in meditation are caused by the method of meditation (Torrey 2001).

Some people see a teacher and follow their meditation

technique for a time; then they read something in some book and decide to try that technique, or a week later they decide to follow some ideas of another famous meditation master. In this way, they may create confusion. Inconsistent use of a meditation technique may not be in an individual's best interest.

Norman E. Rosenthal authored a book (2011) about the benefits of meditation. *Transcendence*, Here Rosenthal promotes that the practice of meditation with people diagnosed with mental illness, such as bipolar disorder and schizophrenia, should be done in conjunction with medication and therapy. It is also important that meditation be monitored and instructed by a professional and only upon the advice of a physician. Norman asserts that this is a balanced approach to apply meditation, and this is the way through which people can manage the symptoms of mental illness in a successful and effective way (Rosenthal 2011).

In considering the effects of relaxation response training on attention deficits in schizophrenia patients, Antonio and Peacock (1988) conducted a small research study of four groups, each consisting of six male patients. Twelve patients were diagnosed with schizophrenia and twelve with antisocial personality disorder. The diagnosis of the diseases was done on the basis of a one-hour unstructured interview and a review of the medical history of the patient. The available information was gathered by a licensed psychologist and an attending physician, as per the criteria mentioned in DSM-III.

To meet the selection criteria, candidates had to be between eighteen and thirty-five years old, selected randomly, and residing in twelve-hundred-bed state hospitals. All the subjects selected were right-handed males with either good or partially good vision. The patients were also prescribed neuroleptic medications. One group out of each category was subjected to diagnostic category, and the other was instructed as the placebo group. After training the groups, they were exposed to an attention task in which they were instructed to manually respond to visual stimuli.

A number of studies have been conducted in the past fifteen years to report the effects of meditation and relaxation upon regulating various aggressive and uncontrollable behaviors. Meditation and relaxation have proven helpful in cases where patients need to develop attention control under nonclinical practices. This study was conducted with the same purpose to examine the effects of meditation and relaxation techniques on attention responses in schizophrenics. One group for individuals with diagnosed schizophrenia group and one group for individuals diagnosed with antisocial personality group received training in Benson's relaxation response under the supervision of a trained technician. The remaining two control groups were only briefed about relaxation and stress management by a trained technician. Both groups were also informed about the general meditation and relaxation process. Immediately after the relevant instructions were delivered to them, the relaxation groups were handed over to another technician to practice the technique to ensure that the initial instructions were well understood. All the instructors involved in the research were blind to the patient diagnosis and history.

Participants were then escorted to laboratory by an experimenter who had no past information of the patients' diagnosis, history, and treatment. After the orientation and adjustment period of fifteen minutes, the relaxation group at Bensons was asked to practice another relaxation response for an additional fifteen minutes. The subjects were than given an experimental task in which three randomly timed red flashlights, located two feet in front of the subject, were presented for a total of five minutes. The variable interval was from one to three seconds, for a total of twenty continuous trials. Each participant was asked to respond to the light by pressing corresponding buttons fixed on a metal box placed on their laps. The correct response was recorded when the subject pressed the matching red flashing button before the next light flashed. An initial practice period allowed the participants to get familiar with the procedure, apparatus, and assessment technique.

Analysis of variance showed no significant difference in the responses of four groups recorded. The type of the disorder, the difference between the instructions, and the practice session did not make any significant changes in the results. However, the practicing of a simple relaxation process did not improve the attention of participants. The study also lacked the baseline data of pretreatment measure, and later a similar study was conducted with a large group to yield a better change in the attention of the treatment groups (Puente and Peacock 1988).

MEDITATION AND SYMPTOMS OF SCHIZOPHRENIA

oving kindness meditation is a kind of meditation that supports the practice of bare attention and helps to keep the mind open with positive thoughts. It also kills negativity and provides ways to support and balance the insight of the meditation we practice. It is a fact that many people in life are troubled by different emotional states, which pressurize them. We live in societies, but we do not have enough skills to deal with the problems societies present. At times, it becomes out of our mind and thoughts to cope with the adjustment mechanism and within others capacity. To let our minds functions properly, we need to develop positive feelings with an essence of sweetness. Loving kindness is a meditation practice taught by Buddha. This practice aims to develop the mental habit of altruistic love and selflessness. Thoughts must be based upon loving kindness, as hatred cannot exist along with it. Loving kindness brings positive changes in attitude, as it systematically develops the state of being loved and improves quality of life. It can also be termed as type of psychotherapy, a way of healing the troubled mind from thoughts that create confusion and pain. Of all the types of Buddhist meditations, loving kindness immediately benefits the mind by changing negative thought patterns into more positive ones. Loving kindness is series of meditations that produce four qualities of love: compassion (*karuna*), friendliness (metta), equanimity (upekkha), and appreciative joy (*mudita*).

Individuals who suffer from the negative symptoms of schizophrenia are most likely to suffer from the disease and represent a subgroup of approximately 15–20 percent (Buchanan 2007). Those who suffer from negative symptoms are prone to decreased response from the treatment. This is because the negative symptoms lead to poorer long-term prognosis and functioning disabilities. The reported negative symptoms comprise five specific symptoms, including blunted affect, avolition, alogia, asociality, and anhedonia. Symptoms like alogia (diminished speech) and blunted affect (diminished expressions of emotion) together represent a single factor. The three remaining factors, asociality (little or no interest in interpersonal relationships), anhedonia (reduced pleasure), and avolition (less motivation), are all closely related and together form another factor (Brantley and Hanauer 2008).The net result of these effects is reduced interest in the normal activities of life, which creates important deficits in quality of life. Anhedonia can be further divided into impairments in anticipatory pleasures (anticipating a pleasurable experience in the future) and consummatory pleasure (the ability of a person to enjoy something at the moment). Consummatory pleasure is integral to a great extent in people suffering from the negative effects of schizophrenia. Anticipatory pleasure can define motivational deficits which gives a better understanding of the negative symptoms. It is difficult to indulge in any activity when there is no anticipation of enjoyment. Asociability, to some extent, is also related to anticipatory pleasure; similarly, a person who does not feel good about a relationship or does not anticipate any social interactions in the future will not be interested in pursuing that relationship or interaction. Therefore, for the healthcare professional, it is necessary to address the negative symptoms of schizophrenia in order to control the suffering of the patients.

ADVANTAGES OF USING MEDITATION AND RELAXATION INTERVENTIONS

A meta-analysis performed on twenty randomized control trials by Arias et al. (2006) to determine the systematic efficacy of meditation techniques when used to treat medical illness concluded that meditation practices are safe and potentially effective in treating certain types of illness, particularly anxiety mood disorder and non-psychotic mood. However this finding needs to be proven by evidence-based practice on large sample sizes. Meditation techniques help patients cope with medical and psychological problems. Recently, an increase in the use and appeal of meditation has been observed, and the scientific knowledge has been put to practice to help schizophrenia patients overcome their condition through non-medical intervention. The analysis was performed on twenty randomized control trials, comprising 958 subjects, 397 acting as experiment subjects and 561 as control subjects. Strongest efficacy was observed in persons diagnosed with epilepsy, menopausal related depression, and premenstrual syndrome. Benefits were also observed in patients with anxiety disorders, emotional disturbances, autoimmune disease, and neoplastic disorders.

Relief of stress and anxiety is one of the most phenomenal

advantages that meditation and relaxation provide. This is the most accepted benefit of meditation and relaxation, whether we are speaking about individuals with diagnosed schizophrenia or the general public. Many research papers suggest that some clinical advantages can be gained by both concentration and mindfulness meditation. These clinical advantages include decreased stress levels, relief of anxiety, reduction of chronic pain, and management of medical illness (Baer 2003, Kabat-Zinn 2003).

Stress-management meditation is perhaps one of the most effective methods of controlling stress. It regains the organization of our observations, inspirations, and thoughts. Stress-management meditation has a biological mechanism, enabling our bodies to collect sufficient oxygen from the environment to feed our muscles, organs, and tissues. To understand the effectiveness of stress meditation management, we must first be able to manage and understand stress. Stress is a physiological factor that causes both emotional and physical strain. It is a measure that tells us precisely when our mind and body are not ready to cope with external pressure and internal negative reflections. As a result of excessive stress, the muscular system becomes tense, and circumstances seem to get out of our control. This decreases our ability to make clear judgments, and the thought process is affected. Stress brings immense physiological changes to our mind and body. It causes neurons to work beyond their capacity, and the result is increased production of toxins. Stress management enables us to clear these toxins by increasing the concentration of oxygen within the brain cells. It helps us to focus our thoughts, lowers blood pressure, and slows breathing and pulse rate. The net result is that the mind is cleared of the stressful thoughts. It also helps to relax our body's muscles and eliminates the lactic acid that builds up during work. Stress-management meditation also helps us to focus and concentrate. When the mind is in a relaxed state, it enables us to organize our thoughts and manage the process in a more effective manner. A relaxed mind makes more effective decisions, compared to a stressed mind, and this ultimately enhances performance and gives us a better chance to perform well.

Stress-management meditation has also been found to be effective in controlling anger and negative thoughts. These are the circumstances usually faced in times of stress. Meditation itself promotes peace, a sense of calmness, and a state of mind of acceptance and forgiveness. A stressed mind does not allow such thoughts to prevail in the mind or the body; therefore, stress management prevents the mind from unhealthy thoughts.

So far, research has concluded that stress management works as a tonic and has no unwanted side-effects. However, positive side-effects have been associated with stress-management meditation. It enriches our lives with fruitful thoughts, wonderful feelings of contentment, and the warmth of life. The key to stress management is visualizing and imaging techniques that promote relaxation. These provide an excellent foundation to perceiving positive thoughts. Such positive aspects are required to overcome difficult situations in life. Stress-management meditation facilitated by a trained professional can improve an individual's overall quality of life.

A simple and easy stress-meditation exercise for ten minutes daily can help us control our depression, anxiety, and cardiovascular health. It gives immense pleasure by increasing the capacity for relaxation. During stress, our body is exposed to sudden biochemical changes. This is characterized as the fight-or-flight response. The mechanism is also referred to as an "adrenaline rush," because the mechanism involves the release of hormones called adrenaline and noradrenalin from the adrenal glands. The excess release of hormones causes an increase in blood pressure, causing increased heart rate, increase blood flow to the muscles, and faster breathing. The meditation or relaxation process elicits the body toward a state of deep relaxation to oppose the fight-or-flight response. Training our bodies in such a way daily achieves a state of wellbeing, enhanced mood, lower blood pressure, and reduction in stress produced by work and life.

IMPROVEMENT IN QUALITY OF LIFE

Overall, quality of life improves when an individual continuously practices meditation. Studies conducted about the usefulness of meditation present primary findings that meditation increases quality of life. Many people have reported that regardless of the symptoms, they feel happy and they do not bother about symptoms. A very precise and comprehensive statement is posited in a research study, which asserts that for individuals diagnosed with schizophrenia, meditation cannot be considered as a cure, but it can definitely help people to feel happy, to move on, and to embrace the courage to deal with their disorder. This research about the use of meditation and relaxation mentions another intriguing factor: just as cardiac patients are advised to do exercise exactly according to the instructions of physicians, individuals diagnosed with schizophrenia must also meditate under the close supervision of a mental health provider or under the guidance of an experienced meditation teacher (Sara 2012).

Daily meditation helps improve quality of life by reducing anxiety and depression. A new research analysis published by Rick Nauert (2014) suggests that meditation provides relief against stress, anxiety, and depression and works as an antidepressant therapy. The new *John Hopkins Review* has published that thirty minutes of meditation daily helps many patients to alleviate chronic and severe anxiety and depression. According to Madhav Goyal, in a study published in *JAMA Internal Medicine*, "Many people use meditation, but this practice is not considered as the mainstream medical therapy for any ailment." But a similar study conducted for the same purpose showed a remarkable decrease in the symptoms of stress and anxiety, dating that meditation provides relief from such symptoms. The therapy is found to function as an antidepressant. Such patients are diagnosed with mixed symptoms of stress, anxiety, and depression, and all these factors contribute toward poor quality of life. Researchers are also working to determine the extent to which these symptoms change the medical and physiological health of a person.

Goyal and his colleagues found that practicing meditation alleviates the symptoms of stress and anxiety. The findings were also compared to those of the placebo effects. During placebo, patients feel better even if they are not receiving any kind of active treatment, as long as they have the perception that they are getting the treatment against ailment they have. To conduct an overview of the research, investigators worked on forty-seven clinical trials performed during the month of June 2013, involving 3,515 participants involved in any kind of meditation practices for various mental illness, such as depression, stress, anxiety, insomnia, substance abuse, and even cardiac problems. The result was a moderate to low level of improvement in the symptoms of depression and anxiety among those participants who went for the eight-week training program of mindfulness meditation. However, for patients suffering from severe symptoms, they did not find any strong evidence of improvement after eight weeks of training. For such patients, it was recommended to follow them up to six months to assess overall improvement or decline. They also concluded that while the patients did not show any improvement from the meditation, neither did they receive any harm.

A misconception about meditation is that one must simply sit down, relax, and do nothing. According to Goyal, this is not true; meditation is a way to actively treat your mind on they ways to increase awareness, and different types of meditations have different approaches. Among many types mindfulness, meditation shows the most promising results when practiced for thirty to forty minutes daily. This type of meditation tunes the mind to accept feelings and thoughts without any kind of judgment and relaxes the mind and body. "Meditation programs appear to have the effect which is above and beyond the placebo," says Goyal (Nauert 2014).

Patients with major depressive disorders (MDD) have a limited quality of life. This is because they cannot overcome the depression, anxiety, and stress from which they usually suffer. QOL assessment and improvement have recently been given importance and are considered an important aspect of healthcare management in general, and for mental disorder patients in particular. In research conducted by William Ishak et al. (2011) to determine the QOL in the patients with MDD, they found that QOL is greatly affected by depression. The degree of depression is also a major contributor in the reduction of QOL; when it is more severe, quality of life is reduced. Depression is considered to be a comorbid condition that exists with psychiatric disorders like schizophrenia and other medical pathologies. The standardized treatment of MDD shows improvement in QOL only in the acute phase, but QOL does remain low when compared with that of normal, healthy individuals. Therefore, it suggested that every physician must include a QOL assessment as an important part of treating depression, anxiety, and stress. Improvement in QOL is an ultimate measure of the success of the treatment.

A study conducted by Yunesian et al. (2008) purports that meditation can be beneficial for people who are suffering from mental illness. When meditation and relaxation techniques are applied for the individuals diagnosed with schizophrenia, they are placed in a meditative state. Being in meditated state helps individuals diagnosed with schizophrenia stay calm and stray away from their hallucinations and illogical thoughts (Yunesian et al. 2008).

It has also been shown that people who experience meditation over a longer period show decreased activity in certain areas of the brain, called the default mode network.

This is the part of the brain that creates lapses in attention as well as disorders like anxiety, hyperactivity, and buildup of beta amyloidal plaques, leading to Alzheimer's disease. The decreased activity of this network is directly related to the performance of the medial prefrontal and posterior cingulated cortex, and this is observed in all kinds of experienced meditators, regardless of the type of meditation they perform. An analysis of the brain scans of the people with increased activity in the default mode network also indicates that meditators constantly monitor and suppress the appearance and emergence of "me" thoughts, also known as mind-wandering. In pathological terms, these states show a direct relationship with diseases like schizophrenia and autism. According to researchers, meditators who developed a new default mode are more present with centered awareness and less self-centered. Experienced meditators' brain scans also show how the areas of the brain associated with schizophrenia, wandering thoughts, psychiatric disorders, and anxiety are switched off.

Meditation is a millennia-old practice to help people to stay in contemplative and philosophical practice. Conversely, it has been verified by many researchers that mental illness in any form is due to a preoccupation with one's own thoughts, and this is primary condition that is affected by meditation. This fact gives us a clear clue as to how neural mechanism are affected clinically in terms of meditation. Therefore, individuals who practice regular meditation are able to control the brain patterns and the functions of the brain. Meditation helps the brain to generate increased and coordinated connectivity between the default mode network and cognitive pathways. This results in optimal brain control. A ruminating brain, which has less coordinated activity between cognitive pathways, is more likely to be associated with depression, attention deficit disorder, and mental illness.

INSTILL A SENSE
OF ACCEPTANCE

Another advantage of applying meditation and relaxing technique is that it is reported to instill a sense of acceptance and sense of belongingness. When individuals with diagnosed schizophrenia are recommended to engage in meditation and relaxation techniques, it is most often within a group setting. Group setting can instill a sense of belonging [to a particular group]. (David et al. 2009).

A widespread practice to develop focus is to place attention on the movement of the breath. Creating focus on one single object prevents our mind from thinking about the rest, and our mind is not occupied by other thoughts. Concentrating on one thing may develop a feeling of peace, comfort, and relaxation. This is how we achieve a state of stability, calmness, and relaxation within our minds.

A systematic review of 144 studies published in the *Journal of Clinical Psychology* clearly states that meditation is better than other available techniques at reducing anxiety by attaining a peaceful mind. It reduces depression, emotional instability, and hostility, and it promotes a more stable, resilient, and balanced personality. In another review of forty-two independent research papers, meditation was found to be effective against a negative mental state by enhancing the state of self-actualization, which is an overall measure of positive mental health and personal development. The three separate and independent components of this are resilient sense of self, positive integrated thinking about life and the world, and emotional maturity.

DISADVANTAGES OF USING MEDITATION AND RELAXATION INTERVENTIONS TO TREAT INDIVIDUALS DIAGNOSED WITH LONG TERM SCHIZOPHRENIA

The use of meditation and relaxation techniques with individuals diagnosed with schizophrenia remains controversial. While limited there are practitioners and researchers that suggest meditation and relaxation techniques can have a negative impact on individuals diagnosed with schizophrenia. The following section discusses some of the disadvantages of using meditation and relaxation techniques to treat individuals diagnosed with schizophrenia.

Adverse Effects of Meditating in Group

There is limited research that provides evidence of the negative impact of meditation. One study purports that meditation may deteriorate the mental condition of a schizophrenic patient. The research points out that meditation represses emotional content. (Varma 2009). However, the research also mentions that in cases where proper guidance by a meditation teacher is present in the process of meditation, relaxation may extract a positive result (Varma 2009).

Another reported disadvantage of meditation for

long-term individuals diagnosed with schizophrenia is that this exercise of meditation or relaxation may precipitate a psychotic episode. According to Roche (2011), during the exercise of meditation, different disturbing experiences, such as anxiety, anger, and tension may be encountered by an individual. As a result, Roche (2011) purports that an individual who has a history of schizophrenia may suffer from a psychotic episode.

There are multiple limitations to the evidence in support or against the use of medication and relaxation with persons diagnosed with long term schizophrenia. Most often in the reviewed studies, variations among these factors have generally been neglected not taking into account the distinctions of age, gender and culture.

THE METHODOLOGY

My research methodology gatheringed relevant data to arrive at a better and logical understanding of how meditation and relaxation are beneficial for long-term individuals diagnosed with schizophrenia. The intention was to answer two questions:

1. Can individuals diagnosed with long-term schizophrenia actively participate in a forty to forty five minute meditation group without being unduly distracted?

2. Can individuals diagnosed with long-term schizophrenia follow the directions given by a facilitator in a guided meditation and be "present in the moment"?

QUALITATIVE AND QUANTITATIVE RESEARCH

B oth quantitative and qualitative data were collected. The priority focus of the analysis was on qualitative outcomes to better understand the benefits gained by the participants. The collected data was evaluated and then analyzed to fully understand the implications of meditation and relaxation on individuals diagnosed with schizophrenia, when incorporated into their treatment milieu, and to determine if there is sufficient evidence to support the claim that meditation and relaxation should be incorporated in the patients' therapy.

Questionnaire as Survey Tool

A questionnaire was utilized to measure attitudes and beliefs of sampled clinical professionals regarding their views and opinions on incorporating meditation and relaxation into the treatment of individuals diagnosed with long term schizophrenia. Questionnaire participants were briefed on the subject matter of incorporating meditation and relaxation into the the treatment milieu of individuals diagnosed with long term schizophrenia. This survey was distributed during the multiple American Counseling Association (ACA) conferences.

The advantages of using a questionnaire are many: it is cost effective, the analysis is simplifed, and it reduces the opportunity for bias. It is also considered to be less intrusive than other survey methods. The responses are collected in a standardized manner, and more than one objective can be followed from the interview results.

One of the survey questions particularly relevant to this study attempts to solicit from participants the length of time that a session (with patients) should last. Participants were asked to choose from among three time periods, fifteen, thirty, and forty-five minutes. The length of time that patients participatinge in a session is of paramount importance, since individuals diagnosed with long term schizophrenia often are also diagnosed with attention deficit disorder.

1. Do you believe individuals diagnosed with long term schizophrenia can actively participate in a meditation and relaxation group? Please circle YES or NO.

a. YES
b. NO

2. If you answered YES, how long do you think they can participate? Please select one of the following:

a. 15 minutes   b. 30 minutes   c. 45 minutes

3. If you answered YES to # 1 above, do you believe that meditation and relaxation can be an adjunct to the inpatients treatment milieu? Please circle YES or NO

a. YES
b. NO

4. If you answered NO to #1 above can you explain why meditation and relaxation should not be incorporated in the patients' therapy?

**THANK YOU FOR PARTICIPATING
IN THIS SURVEY**

RESPONDENTS
OF THE STUDY

analyzed the responses from ninety-three randomly selected clinical professionals, most of whom practiced in behavioral health. Questionnaires were distributed to participants over a four-year period. The sampled population of participants identified as doctors of philosophy, psychologists, licensed mental health counselors, registered professional nurses, and mental health nurses.

Participants were randomly chosen with the majority of responders being attendees at the American Counseling Association Conferences held in North Carolina in 2009, Pennsylvania in 2010, Louisiana in 2011, and California in 2012. These clinical professionals who participated in the survey were knowledgeable with the disease concept of individuals diagnosed with long term schizophrenia. They identified as being well versed on the subject of meditation and relaxation as a treatment component for individuals diagnosed with long term schizophrenia. The survey aimed to collect information on the beliefs and attitudes of these professionals and to obtain input as to whether it is their experience that individuals diagnosed with long term schizophrenia could benefit from meditation and relaxation therapy, if added to their therapy milieu.

RESULTS AND DISCUSSION

There was 95.6 percent response rate (leaving only a non-response rate of only 4.4 percent). The relatively small non-response group included out-of-state participants, who rationalized that, as students in the field of behavioral health, they had limited experience with individuals diagnosed with schizophrenia and could not participate in the study.

The eighty-six responding questionnaire participants were from different states, as previously indicated; however, they were professionally grouped, starting with the highest level of their education. The following table illustrates the professional level of the participants, their responses, and the chosen length of time that patients should participate in the meditation and relaxation group. They selected a length of time from among three given choices: fifteen, thirty, or forty-five minutes.

CHARLOTTE (2009), PITTSBURGH (2010), NEW ORLEANS (2011), SAN FRANCISCO (2012)			
SPECIALIZATION	EDUCATIONAL LEVEL	RECOMMENDED PARTICIPATION TIME BY NUMBERS	
		45 minutes	30 minutes
Behavioral health	PhD	20	5
Multicultural counselors & advocates	PhD	5	0
Family counselor educator	PhD	2	1
Counselor educator	PhD	7	5
Registered clinical Educator in mental health	MS	15	10
HUDSON VALLEY. MONTROSE HOSPITAL ENVIRONS			
Doctors	PhD	5	0
Licensed mental health counselors		3	0
Registered professional psychiatric nurses		12	0

Note: No participants selected 15 minutes.

Analysis of the Results

The first group comprised the twenty-five behavioral health PhD participants, twenty of whom indicated a preference for the forty-five-minute period, while five showed a preference for the thirty-minute period. The second group consisted of five PhD multicultural counselors and advocates. They also expressed a preference for forty-five minutes, while out of the third group of three PhD family counselor educators, two showed a preference for forty-five minutes, and the other group member indicated a preference for thirty minutes. From among the fourth group, consisting of twelve PhD counselor educators, seven expressed a preference for forty-five minutes, while five preferred the thirty-minute period. The fifth group consisted of twenty-five registered clinical counselors in mental health with master's level of education, and of this group, fifteen showed a preference for forty-five minutes, while the remaining ten preferred a thirty-minute period. No information was obtained from the sixth and final group of three PhD students, who rationalized that they lacked adequate experience to weigh in on the subject. Additionally, sixteen other healthcare professional, including three PhD, two licensed mental health counselors (LMHC), and eleven registered professional nurses who had been working in the mental health field for about fifteen years, around the Hudson Valley area including Montrose Veteran's Administration Hospital, participated in the study. All demonstrated a preference for the forty-five-minute time period.

The results of the study indicate that 78 percent of all PhDs favor the forty-five-minute duration, while only 22 percent favor the thirty-minute duration. Among professionals with a master's, the difference between those who showed a preference for the forty-five- and thirty-minute duration is less, 60 percent and 40 percent respectively. From among professionals with less than a master's degree, 100 percent favored the forty-five-minute period. It also should be noted that 100 percent of all professionals in the New York area favor the forty-five-minute duration for meditation and relaxation. None of the surveyed participants favor a fifteen-minute during for the meditation and relaxation group.

The duration of subjects' participation in the meditation and relaxation program appears to be of concern for some of the surveyed participants. For example, one of the participants who selected the thirty-minute duration commented that thirty minutes should be adequate for the patients with a diagnosis of schizophrenia, because their attention span can be very short", while another offered the following: "Most times individuals diagnosed with schizophrenia are responding to internal stimuli. Attending a meditation and relaxation group by this population should last for thirty minutes." Another participant who preferred the forty-five-minute duration offered the following: "Depending on the level of functioning of the patients, they probably can participate in the meditation and relaxation group for forty-five minutes or more."

From the data, it is quite plausible that the vast number of PhD professionals who favor the forty-five-minute duration for the meditation and relaxation group might be aware that some individuals diagnosed with schizophrenia will show mild to moderate disorganization and episodic paranoia that does not affect their functioning stability. There is also the possible explanation that the patients, though being diagnosed with schizophrenia, have less profound functional impairment and confusion associated with their mental illness. These two factors quite likely explain their rationale for weighing in so heavily in favor of a forty-five-minute period for participation in the meditation and relaxation group. It should be noted that surveyed participants favored a thirty- or forty-five-minute period, while none opted for the fifteen-minute duration. This is a significant finding since patients' participation time is one of the key factors in my study. Also, from among survey participants, there was strong evidence that a meditation and relaxation group, if added to the treatment milieu of the chronic individuals diagnosed with schizophrenia, would be of significant benefit to the patients.

CONCLUSION

The results of the questionnaire affirmed that a meditation and relaxation group could be added to the treatment milieu of individuals diagnosed with long term schizophrenia and benefits could be expected from participation in the group. The vast majority of respondents showed a preference for forty-five minutes for clients to participate in a meditation and relaxation group. None of the surveyed participants opted for the fifteen-minute duration.

This study shows evidence that individuals diagnosed with long term schizophrenia can benefit from participation in a meditation and relaxation group. This study can raise awareness among most behavioral health providers that meditation and relaxation can be incorporated in the treatment of individuals diagnosed with long term schizophrenia in both hospital and private practice settings.

PATIENT CASE STUDIES

The following case studies are described to show the clinical feasibility, challenges, and diagnoses of individuals with long term schizophrenia. Assessment of the psychiatric disorder, emotions, symptoms, and recovery was conducted at the baseline, pretreatment, posttreatment, and three-month follow-up levels after the treatment. Patients belonged to different age groups, from young adults to middle age, and were included because of a primary diagnosis of schizophrenia. All the patients were on antipsychotic medicines during the course of therapy. The intervention took place in a group setting. Each session was conducted by a mental health therapist with over twenty-five years experience in meditation. With informed participant consent they were asked questions about their medical history, diagnosis, and state of mind before and after the meditation sessions. Participants were advised that all information shared would be maintained as confidential.

The following sample Participant experiences are symbolic of most participant outcomes.

Participant One

Participant One is a single, young adult female, diagnosed with schizophrenia and associated anxiety disorder. She identifies as African-American. She presented with symptoms of uneasiness; she had difficulty interacting with people around her, was not able to pay attention, and was always evaluating herself negatively. Participant One had been in psychotherapy for the previous one year before she started participating in the meditation therapy. Participant One initially did not respond well and reported that others were evaluating her negatively. However, her assessment before and after the session showed marked improvement in positive emotions and a decrease in unpleasant emotions. With regular practicing, she also started actively participating in the group discussion.

Participant Two

Participant Two is a middle-aged woman, living with her parents, siblings and husband. Prior to joining the meditation group, she expressed concern about the level of conversation she would have to participate in. Despite her concerns she hesitantly joined the group for the purpose of meditation. She initially had difficulty in the group, reporting racing thoughts. The trainer guided her in individual sessions with specific excercises to decrease the anxiety and racing thoughts. Over time, Participant Two came to prefer group sessions and no longer was distracted during the group session.

Participant Three

Participant Three was an adult male in his early thirties living with his family as a single man. His parents suggested that he join the meditation group. He had always faced difficulty in recreational activities and maintaining employment. Upon joining the meditation group, Participant Three was often silent even when addressed. With instruction he started practicing meditation and relaxation techniques independently two to three times a day for periods of ten minutes. After a period of weeks, his weekly and post-assessment reports suggested improvements in his negative symptoms of asociality, flat affect, alogia, and avolition. He also reported that meditation made him feel relaxed and that mindful breathing helped him cover his negative auditory hallucinations.

REFERENCES

Alexander, C. N., K. G. Walton, and D. W. Johnson. 2013. "Preventing Disasters and Distress through the Transcendental Meditation and TM-Sidhi Program." In *Consciousness Based Government*, MUM Press.

Arias, A. J., K. Steinberg, A. Banga, and R. L. Trestman. 2006. "Systematic Review of the Efficacy of Meditation Techniques as Treatments for Medical Illness." *Journal of Alternative & Complementary Medicine* 12(8): 817–832. http://online.liebertpub.com/doi/abs/10.1089/acm.2006.12.817.

Baumeister, R. F., and, M. R. Leary. 1995. "The Need to Belong: Desire for Interpersonal Attachments As a Fundamental Human Motivation." *Psychological Bulletin* 117: 497–529.

Beckwith, M. 2008. "Reclaim Your Power. Super Change Your Life." http://senseitristan.wordpress.com/2008/01/10/michael-beckwith-on-meditation/.

Beckwith, M. B. 2008. *Spiritual Liberation: Fulfilling Your Soul's Potential.* New York: Atria Books.

Benson, H. 1976. *The Relaxation Response*. New York: William Morrow & Co, Inc.

Bogart, G. (1991). The use of meditation in psychotherapy: A review of the literature. *American Journal of Psychotherapy, 45*(3), 383-412. http//www.dawnmountain.com/artmordernpsyc,htmlhotherapy.

Brantley, M., T. Hanauer. 2008. *The Gift of Loving-kindness: 100 Meditations on Compassion, Generosity, and Forgiveness*. Oakland: New Harbinger Publications.

Brown, K. W., R. M. Ryan. 2003. "The Benefits of Being Present: Mindfulness and Its Role in Psychological Well-Being." *Journal of Personality and Social Psychology* 84(4): 822. http://psycnet.apa.org/journals/psp/84/4/822/.

Brown, C., and A. Jones. 2010. "Meditation Experience Predicts Less Negative Appraisal of Pain: Electrophysiological Evidence for the Involvement of Anticipatory Neural Responses."

Brown, P. N. 2010. "Easing Ills through Tai Chi." *Harvard Magazine* (January- February).

Buchanan, R. W. 2007. "Persistent Negative Symptoms in Schizophrenia: An Overview." *Schizophrenia Bulletin* 33(4): 1013–1022.

Deatherage, G. 1975. "The Clinical Use of Mindfulness Meditation Techniques in Short-Term Therapy." *Journal of Transpersonal Psychology*. Issue 2.

Deikman, A. 1982. *The Observing Self: Mysticism and Psychotherapy*. Beacon Press. http://www.depression-solutions.com/insight-answers/dopamine.

DSM-IV. 1994. *Diagnostic and Statistical Manual of Mental Disorders*, 4th ed. American Psychiatric Association.

Hick, S. F., and T. Bien. 2008. *Mindfulness and the Therapeutic Relationship*. New York: Guilford Press.

Holden, L. 2010. *QI Healing: Energy Practices for Health & Vitality*. DVD. Boulder: Sounds True, Inc.

Ishak, W. W., J. M. Greenberg, K. Balayan, N. Kapitanski, J. Jeffrey, H. Fathy and M. H. Rapaport. 2011. "Quality of Life: the Ultimate Outcome Measure of Interventions in Major Depressive Disorder." Harvard Review of Psychiatry 19(5): 229–239. http://informahealthcare.com/doi/abs/10.3109/10673229.2011.614099.

Johnson, D. W. 2006. "Evidence that the Transcendental Meditation Program Prevents or Decreases Diseases of the Nervous System and Is Specifically Beneficial for Epilepsy." *Medical Hypotheses*. Issue 2.

Lindberg, D. A. 2005. "Integrative Review of Research Related to Meditation, Spirituality, and the Elderly." *Geriatric Nursing* 26(6): 372–77. http://www.sciencedirect.com/science/article/pii/S0197457205003794.

Luzader, Cheynne, and Kevin Roth. 2002. *Guided Imagery for Stress Release and Relaxation*. CD. Hollywood, Florida: Star Gazer Studios.

Mitchell, R. L. C., R. Elliott, M. Barry, et al. 1995. "The Neural Response to Emotional Prosody, As Revealed by Functional Magnetic Resonance Imaging." *Neuro-psychologia*.

Mitchell, S. A., M. J. Black. 1995. *Freud and Beyond: A History of Modern Psychoanalytic Thought*.

Nauert, R. 2014. "Daily Meditation Helps with Mild-Moderate Anxiety, Depression." *Psych Central*. http://psychcentral. com/news/2014/01/08/daily-meditation-helps-with-mild-moderate-anxiety-depression/64233.html.

Publication manual of the American Psychological Association 5th ed. American Association - American Psychological Association – 2007.

Puente, E. A., and A. L. Peacock. 1988. "Effects of Relaxation Response Training on Attentional Deficits in Schizophrenics." *Perceptual and Motor Skills* 66: 789–90. http://antonioepuente.com/wp-content/uploads/2013/01/1988.-Effects-of-relaxation-response-training-on-attentional-deficits-in-schizophrenia-1988.pdf.

Rosenthal, N.E. 2011. *Transcendence: Healing and Transformation through Transcendental Meditation*. Penguin Group.

Rubia, K. 2009. "The Neurobiology of Meditation and Its Clinical Effectiveness in Psychiatric Disorders." *Biological Psychology* 82: 1–11. http://www.sciencedirect.com/ science/article/pii/S0301051109000775.

Shapiro, S., et al. 2008. "Mechanisms of Mindfulness." *Journal of Clinical Psychology*. Issue 7.

Soanes, C. *Oxford Dictionary of Current English*, 3rd ed. Oxford: Oxford University Press.

Spearing, M. K., et al. 1999. "Overview of different types of Schizophrenia." *National Institutes of Mental Health*. 413–23.

Tang, Y. Y., Y. Ma, J. Wang, Y. Fan, S. Feng, Q. Lu, and M. I. Posner. 2007. "Short-Term Meditation Training Improves Attention and Self-Regulation." *Proceedings of the National Academy of Sciences* 104(43): 17152–56. http://www.pnas.org/content/104/43/17152.short.

Tipping, C. 2009. *Radical Forgiveness.* Boulder: Sounds True.

Yunesian, M., Aslani, A., Vash, J., & Yazdi, A. (2008). Effects of Transcendental Meditation on mental health: a before-after study. *Clinical Practice and Epidemiology in Mental Health, 4*(1), 25. doi:10.1186/1745-0179-4-25